Understandir

BLOOL
PRESSURE

Professor Alan J. Silman

Published by Family Doctor Publications Limited
in association with the British Medical Association

IMPORTANT

This book is intended to supplement the advice given to you by your doctor. The author and publisher have taken every care in its preparation. In particular, information about drugs and dosages has been thoroughly checked. However, before taking any medication you are strongly advised to read the product information sheet accompanying it. Your pharmacist will be able to help you with anything you do not understand.

© Family Doctor Publications 1993, 1995
Reprinted 1994
Second edition 1995
Reprinted 1996
Medical Editor: Dr Tony Smith
Cover Artist: Colette Blanchard
Illustrator: Angela Christie
Design: Create Publishing Services Ltd., Bath
Printing: Reflex Litho Ltd, using acid-free paper

ISBN: 1 898205 05 1

Contents

The Surgery
High Street
Anytown

Date as postmark

Dear Mrs Dunningham

We have just been reviewing the medical records of our patients who have recently had their fortieth birthday. We note that you have not had your blood pressure checked recently.

As this would be useful, we suggest you make an appointment to see one of us. The whole procedure won't take very long and we can discuss the benefits of your having this check up when you come along to the surgery.

Yours sincerely

W. B. O'Brian

pp. The Doctors

Introduction

Many of us will receive a letter similar to the one opposite from our family doctor, often on reaching the age of 35 or 40. Some will be pleased at this opportunity to check that all is well: others may view it indignantly as yet another unwelcome reminder that they are getting older, and would prefer not to think about it.

The following pages should, we hope, confirm the view of those in the former group and help those in the latter group understand why it is important to have their blood pressure checked.

This booklet takes the form of fictitious consultations between a patient with high blood pressure and his general practitioner and encompasses the many questions asked by those with this condition.

What is blood pressure?

● Could you tell me what blood pressure is?

Blood pressure is the force with which the heart pumps blood through the arteries and so allows the blood to reach the various parts of the body. Without this pressure the blood would not flow sufficiently to be able to supply the body with the necessary oxygen and food. When people lose a lot of blood, perhaps after a bad accident, the heart has much less to pump and the pressure drops dramatically – a state called 'shock'.

● So does the blood pressure depend on how much blood the heart pumps out?

In part this is so. The blood pressure is related to the amount of blood pumped out of the heart with each beat. However, you may remember from physics at school that if the same volume of liquid has to be pumped through a narrow pipe there will be greater pressure in that pipe than if the pipe were wider. In the body, these pipes through which the blood is pumped – the arteries – can actually alter their width, particularly in the small arteries in the skin and muscles. The tighter these are shut, the greater the blood pressure. This can sometimes be very useful. For example, after a major road traffic accident with a lot of bleeding, if the blood vessels in the skin and muscles close down it means that there is sufficient blood pressure to ensure that the blood reaches the important organs, such as the heart and brain.

● Some people say they have 'low blood pressure'. Does this mean that they go dizzy and faint a lot?

There are a few, rare medical conditions associated with an abnormally low blood pressure, but more often, when doctors refer to low blood pressure, they mean it is normal!

Their main concern is with high blood pressure, and they may reassure a patient with normal blood pressure by telling him or her that it is low.

● Is it the blood pressure that you feel when you take the pulse at the wrist?
Yes. With each heartbeat the blood pressure varies.

It is at its highest when the heart is pumping out the blood, and at its lowest when it is filling up again. So when we measure blood pressure we have to record two pressure readings – the highest known as the systolic, and the lowest, the diastolic. It is the rise and fall of blood pressure with each cycle of the heartbeat that produces the wave felt on taking the pulse.

● Can you tell the actual level of blood pressure by feeling the pulse?
Not really. It is usually impossible to tell whether a person has high or normal blood pressure by feeling their pulse, although in the case of shock, which is mentioned above, the pulse is very thin and may be extremely difficult to feel.

KEY POINTS

✓ Blood has to be under pressure to reach all parts of the body

✓ High blood pressure is frequently a problem; low blood pressure rarely is

✓ Blood pressure rises as the heart pumps out blood, and falls as it fills up again

✓ The rise and fall creates the pressure wave we can feel as a pulse

Measuring blood pressure

● How is blood pressure measured?

By using a machine called a sphygmomanometer. However this measures it indirectly. The actual pressure inside the arteries can only be determined by putting a pressure gauge of some sort inside the artery. (This is sometimes done, but mainly for research purposes.) For all practical purposes the sphygmomanometer is perfectly satisfactory, and works by measuring the pressure wave of the pulse.

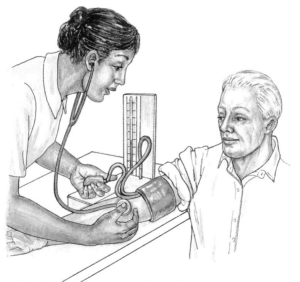

Blood pressure is measured with a machine called a sphygmomanometer.

How does it work?

First a bandage or cuff is wrapped around the upper arm. Inside this is a bag which can be inflated by squeezing the rubber bulb attached to it by a tube. The bulb has a screw-cap which can be released to deflate the bag. If the bag is inflated to a high enough pressure it will eventually prevent any blood travelling through the arteries to the rest of the arm.

A second tube from the bag goes into the machine and carries the pressure to be measured. This pressure pushes up the column of mercury in the glass tube, which is marked with a scale (which is shown

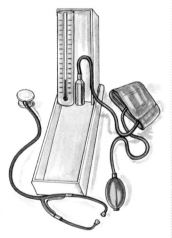

Mercury sphygmomanometer

in millimetres of mercury – mmHg). By reading the height of the mercury column the value for blood pressure can be determined.

What is the actual procedure?

First the bag is pumped up until the blood flow is restricted and a pulse can no longer be felt in the arm: it is then inflated slightly more.

Next, the bag is allowed to deflate slowly and when the pressure in the cuff is equivalent to the maximum, or systolic, pressure blood will again begin to flow.

By placing a stethoscope over the inside of the elbow, it is possible to hear when this happens quite precisely.

As the bag continues to be deflated, the noises continue to be heard until the lowest part of the pulse pressure cycle, the diastolic pressure, is reached, when they cease.

Taking the blood pressure involves noting these two measurements from the mercury column of the sphygmomanometer.

Does it feel uncomfortable?

Pumping air into the cuff is equivalent to squeezing the arm tightly, which may momentarily feel a little uncomfortable. Furthermore, if the blood supply to the hand is cut off temporarily, as happens when the bag is fully inflated, the nerve endings in the fingers feel the lack of blood flow and the finger tips may tingle. As the cuff remains inflated for a short time only, this temporary interruption in blood flow to the arm is not harmful in any way.

● Are there different sorts of sphygmomanometer?

Yes, though the mercury column type is the most common. Some doctors use a more compact one called an aneroid sphygmomanometer, in which the pressure is recorded against normal air resistance, in the same way as a tyre pressure is determined. Thus, instead of the mercury column, there is a clock-face type scale with a pointer. This sort of sphygmomanometer is much lighter and more convenient for home visits, but it is not as accurate as the mercury type.

Electronic machines are becoming very popular because the flow of blood is picked up electronically and measurement does not rely on the human ear and stethoscope. These

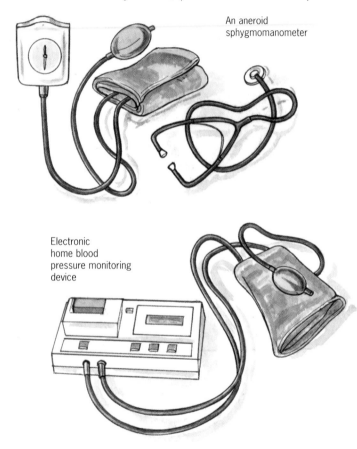

An aneroid sphygmomanometer

Electronic home blood pressure monitoring device

machines are becoming increasingly available and have the advantage that it is possible to measure one's own blood pressure. I have seen them advertised quite a lot recently, though I am not sure that it is a particularly good idea to measure your own blood pressure. More importantly, electronic devices are not necessarily more accurate than conventional mercury types; indeed, it is difficult to better the human ear in its ability to detect and differentiate between various sounds.

● I have seen machines that people can use for recording their own blood pressure in large department stores. Are they a good idea?

Most doctors would be worried about patients checking their own blood pressure in the middle of a long, exhausting shopping expedition!

It is quite possible that the pressure could be raised as a result of shopping and the patient understandably might become unduly alarmed.

A large number of factors can affect blood pressure, and a doctor has to take these into account when interpreting the readings he obtains.

KEY POINTS

✓ Blood pressure is measured in millimetres of mercury (mmHg) by a sphygmomanometer

✓ Both the peak pressure (systolic) and low pressure (diastolic) measurements of the pulse are recorded

✓ DIY measurements are not reliable

What can affect blood pressure?

● Do factors such as anger, stress, fatigue or exercise affect the blood pressure in healthy people?

Blood pressure is affected by emotions, such as fear or anger, but the effect tends to be short-lived.

More importantly, blood pressure varies considerably in any 24-hour period. Not surprisingly, it is at its lowest in the middle of the night and at its peak at the end of a working day. Some of this change is due to normal rhythms in the body's chemistry, but some is probably related to stress and exercise. The difference can be very large, and if you have been diagnosed as having high blood pressure, it is important that you should always have your blood pressure measured at approximately the same time of day, otherwise it might be difficult to decide whether any change was due to treatment or variation in timing.

(Also remember that if you ever need a life insurance medical examination it makes sense to have it early rather than later on in the day!)

Many patients come rushing into the surgery late for their appointment and they should wait and rest for about ten minutes before being checked.

In addition, even 'limited' exercise, such as talking or chewing while the blood pressure is being measured, can put up the reading. Blood pressure can also rise after a large meal.

● Is it really worth measuring blood pressure? It seems to be affected by so many things.

Doctors and others who measure blood pressure take account of the various factors which might affect someone's blood pressure, and recognise the importance of using the same method each time. So most people find that their doctor normally uses the right arm, as there might be a slight difference between the arms; the person is usually seated and the sphygmomanometer is kept at the same level relative to the body.

KEY POINTS

✓ Blood pressure varies naturally over a 24-hour period

✓ Blood pressure can be affected in the short-term by emotions, exercise, stress and eating

Why is high blood pressure important?

● Why are doctors particularly interested in blood pressure when it is high?

Hypertension (the medical term for high blood pressure) is not a disease in itself, but its presence leads to an increased risk of developing some rather serious conditions late in life, such as heart attack and stroke.

In a heart attack, part of the blood supply to the heart becomes blocked and some of the heart muscle can die or 'infarct'. This may weaken the heart's action as a pump or even cause sudden death. Most people who suffer a heart attack make a full recovery, but it is obviously a worrying condition.

Strokes associated with high blood pressure can be one of two types. In the first, the blood supply to a part of the brain gets blocked and that part dies or becomes damaged. In the second, the constant high pressure can cause a small blood vessel to burst and the pressure of this leak can also damage the brain. The major result from either type of stroke is weakness, or possibly paralysis of an arm or leg. Sometimes the whole of one side of the body may be affected, and speech can also be impaired. Fortunately, many patients with a stroke recover completely, often with 24 hours, but for others the weakness may last some months, and for a few it may be permanent.

● How much does high blood pressure increase the risk of these events?

The important thing to remember is that the large majority of those with high blood pressure will not develop these problems. Also, many people with normal blood pressure will suffer heart attacks and strokes too. It is just that the risk of developing them is increased in people with hypertension.

The actual increase in risk

depends on the level of blood pressure (the higher the pressure the higher the risk), and also on age and sex (high blood pressure causes relatively more problems in men and in older people). It is also important to remember that though high blood pressure may increase the chance of a stroke ten times in a 25-year-old man he is more likely to be killed in a car accident in the next ten years than he is to die prematurely because of high blood pressure.

● So is there any point in diagnosing high blood pressure under a certain age?

Many family doctors invite their patients to have their blood pressure checked when they reach the age of 40. Some even advise having this first check at 35 or even 30. Below this there is, under normal circumstances, perhaps little point.

● Is there an upper age limit? For instance, is high blood pressure a risk factor in my mother aged 79?

As I have said, high blood pressure has a greater chance of causing a stroke in a woman aged 79 than in one aged 39. So it could be much more serious for an elderly person to be hypertensive than for a younger person. However, some doctors take the view that high blood pressure is only a 'risk factor' and if one has reached the age of 80 in good health and the blood pressure is raised, then perhaps it is a little unfair to make too many changes to lifestyle or to start taking drug treatment. I think, however, we have become more aware recently of the need to maintain health even into the oldest age group and, yes, we would take your mother's high blood pressure as seriously as somebody who is younger.

KEY POINTS

✓ High blood pressure – hypertension – increases the risk of heart attack and stroke

✓ Risk increases with age, and is higher for men than women

Diagnosing high blood pressure

● You have now taken my blood pressure. Is it high?

The reading is 170/108 mmHg. The two numbers refer respectively to the systolic and diastolic blood pressures discussed earlier on page 7. We have to make some arbitrary decisions as to what might be considered normal/abnormal levels of blood pressure. As a rough rule, a systolic pressure under 140 mmHg and a diastolic pressure under 90 mmHg are normal. The two readings tend to be either low or high together. Figures above 160/100 mmHg are high, and any readings between these and normal levels are considered borderline. If your blood

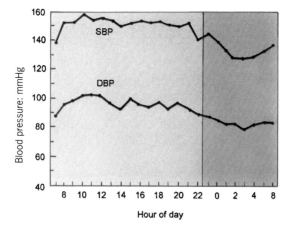

A systolic (peak) blood pressure reading (SBP in the above graph) under 140 mmHg and a diastolic (low) blood pressure reading (DBP) under 90 mmHg are generally regarded as normal.

pressure was in this intermediate range I would only ask you to come back after 12 months and have it checked again.

● So does my reading indicate I have high blood pressure?

No, not necessarily. Remember there are many factors which can affect blood pressure. Anxiety is one of them, and one common source of anxiety is having your blood pressure measured! In fact it is very common for a high reading to drop once you have your blood pressure taken for a second time. I could do another reading today, but a good policy is to repeat the measurement after about a week and, if it is still high, to repeat again after a further four weeks. I only diagnose somebody as having high blood pressure

if it remains high after these three readings. In many people the blood pressure can fall quite dramatically to normal within those few weeks. In others, blood pressure is more variable, changing between normal and higher levels. This is sometimes referred to as labile blood pressure, and with these people it needs checking more regularly, perhaps every six months or so.

● Well, this is my third visit, and my blood pressure is still up. Would you now classify me as a patient with high blood pressure?

Yes, but I should emphasise that your case is not serious. The increase from normal blood pressure is only modest, and as you have now been diagnosed, there is little need to worry.

KEY POINTS

✓ Blood pressure measurements vary from reading to reading

✓ There is no definite cut off for high blood pressure

✓ Most doctors agree that under 140/90 mmHg is normal, and over 160/100 mmHg is high

Discovering high blood pressure

● Although my blood pressure is high, I feel perfectly well. Shouldn't I be suffering from headaches or perhaps some other symptom?

Most people imagine that high blood pressure results in symptoms like headache and dizziness. The truth is that unless it is extremely high it very rarely causes any such problems.

● But I am sure I have heard of people who said that their high blood pressure was discovered after complaining to their doctor about headaches.

This is very possible – both headaches and high blood pressure are common – but it does not mean that the two factors are related. It is much more likely that the doctor took the opportunity to measure their blood pressure when they can to the surgery.

Because of the lack of symptoms, most cases of hypertension would be missed if doctors actually waited for people to come to them.

● Is that why you sent me the letter?

Yes. Most general practitioners now are using this population screening approach in which we actively try and cover all the patients on our list. The only other alternative would have been to wait until you came to the surgery for some other reason, and use that opportunity to measure your blood pressure.

In fact, about 90 per cent of people will have visited their doctor within any three-year period, thus allowing him to check their medical record and measure their blood pressure if there is no recent reading.

Many people have their blood pressure measured as part of a life insurance or work medical examination.

Similarly, attendance at an

ante-natal or family planning clinic is used as an opportunity to detect hypertension in women.

In the United States you are quite likely to have your blood pressure checked by your dentist or even your local pharmacist – so you can see it is getting very difficult to escape the screening net wherever you live!

KEY POINTS

✓ Hypertension is usually symptomless

✓ Most people have their blood pressure regularly checked. If you are over 40 and don't, you should

Causes of high blood pressure

● Can you tell me what causes hypertension?

Unfortunately, we can discover an identifiable cause for the hypertension in only about two or three percent of cases. If this is discovered and treated, the hypertension can actually be cleared up.

I suppose the commonest of these medical causes I see is in patients treated with a group of drugs called steroids. These are used in many disorders, such as asthma and severe arthritis, and, if given in a large enough dose and for a long period of time, can result in hypertension. When the drug is stopped the blood pressure usually returns to normal.

Some women develop high blood pressure in pregnancy but it usually returns to normal afterwards. Hypertension early in pregnancy may indicate a high chance of developing it in later life, but when the pressure rises later in pregnancy (a condition known as pre-eclampsia) it will only recur, if at all, during subsequent pregnancies.

Sometimes people are born with a narrowing of the main artery of the body or have a narrowing of an artery to a kidney. For different and fairly complicated reasons, these anatomical features cause hypertension, but they can be treated surgically. Other causes include rare tumours which produce hormones that increase blood pressure, and these can also be removed surgically. Finally, if a patient has very severe kidney disease from any cause then this may raise the blood pressure. But kidney disease usually shows itself in other ways as well, and for a new, mildly hypertensive patient like yourself with no other symptoms, this is a highly unlikely cause of raised blood pressure.

● You say that it is unlikely that I have any of these rare conditions, but can you be sure?

Not absolutely certain, no, but there are a few simple tests which I carry out in all my new patients with hypertension to rule out these rare causes.

● So what is the cause of hypertension in most patients?

There is unlikely to be a single cause: the high blood pressure is probably the result of a number of factors. Firstly, blood pressure rises with age, though we are not clear about the reasons for this. Since this age-related increase does not always occur in non-Westernised societies, some people believe that hypertension is a disease of Western civilisation.

● Do you mean that this condition is related to stress?

Perhaps, but I suspect that having to search for food during a drought in Africa is just as stressful as commuting to work in London. The problem is that it is very difficult to measure stress. People tend to measure the causes, but it is the individual reaction to events that is important. For example, some people become very tense before exams, while others remain calm. Nevertheless there is no doubt that relaxation can reduce blood pressure, so stress is likely to be of importance in some people. I should emphasise that, within the UK, hypertension is not found to a

greater extent in executives than in manual workers.

● What about diet?

The most obvious aspect of diet is a very strong association between being overweight and hypertension – indeed, obesity is the most important risk factor after age. What is more, we know that if overweight people lose weight, then their hypertension can disappear. If I wanted to reduce the number of people with high blood pressure in this country, my main strategy would be to reduce the extent of obesity.

● Magazines and newspapers are full of the evils of salt – is it important?

Although this is one of the most researched areas, the results are inconclusive. On balance, however, salt probably is important. If all salt-containing foods are cut out of the diet completely, the blood pressure can drop dangerously and produce a state of shock, so salt must be important in maintaining a normal blood pressure. It is also true that hypertension is rare in those countries whose populations have a low salt intake. The northern Japanese, for instance, have a high salt intake and high levels of hypertension, whereas the opposite is found in the south of the country. In Britain, though, no relation has been found

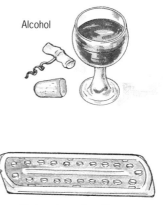
Alcohol

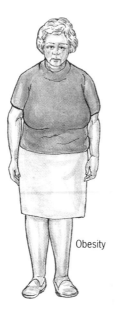
Obesity

Oral contraceptive pill

Smoking

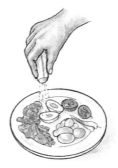
Salt (sodium)

between an individual's salt intake and his or her blood pressure. This does not mean, however, that salt intake is unimportant: one explanation for the disparity is that we British all take too much salt and are therefore all at risk!

● Are there any other important aspects of diet?

A few, but these have not really been proved. Just as a high salt (or to be more precise, sodium), intake may be harmful, it has been suggested that a low intake of potassium, another mineral, may also increase the risk.

Interestingly, sodium and potassium are inversely related to each other in many foods – that is foods high in one are low in the other and vice versa. Natural and fresh foods, for example oranges, are usually high in potassium and low in sodium, whereas processed foods, for example orange cordials, are high in sodium and low in potassium.

● What about smoking and alcohol? They seem to cause everything!

There is some evidence to suggest that smoking can increase the risk of hypertension, though its effect is small compared with, say, body weight.

As a separate issue, however, smoking increases the risk of unpleasant long-term outcomes of hypertension – heart attack and stroke – so it is particularly ill-advised for someone with high blood pressure to smoke.

Alcohol taken in normal quantities probably has little effect on blood pressure, and in small quantities might be beneficial. Moderate, regular drinking does, however, seem to raise the blood pressure.

● Are any other aspects of lifestyle important?

The oral contraceptive pill may cause or precipitate hypertension in some women.

As this is fairly well recognised, women who are taking the pill usually have their blood pressure checked regularly, say, every six months.

● Does hypertension run in families? An aunt of mine has hypertension, so that presumably explains my blood pressure being high.

This is a difficult one, as hypertension is very common. Depending on your definition, it probably affects one in five of the population. So it is highly likely that most people will have one relative with hypertension.

Having said that, there is a close association of hypertension within families.

Children of hypertensive parents tend to have higher, though still normal, blood pressures than children of parents with normal blood pressure. It is also likely that genetic effects explain why some people can eat vast amounts of salt and not have high blood pressure.

It is important to realise that the genetic mechanisms governing the inheritance of hypertension are complicated. Unlike those governing say hair or eye colour, where it is easy to follow the characteristics through the generations, the inheritance of hypertension cannot be predicted with any certainty.

● Are there ethnic differences in blood pressure?

Yes, those of Afro-Caribbean origin, for example, have a high risk of hypertension, but whether this represents a true ethnic effect or whether it reflects differences in lifestyle is difficult to know.

KEY POINTS

✓ Medical causes of hypertension account for 2-3 per cent of cases

✓ Other risk factors for hypertension are:

Genetic factors	+++
Obesity	+++
High sodium intake	++
Contraceptive pill	++
Alcohol	+
Smoking	+
Stress	?

The follow-up consultation

● This is my first proper consultation since you detected high blood pressure. What is the plan now?

First, I must ask some questions. I need to know whether you have any family history of hypertension (in a parent, brother or sister), as this would suggest a genetic link in your developing the condition. I will also ask about possible kidney disease in the past, and information about any drugs you may be taking that could have increased your blood pressure (though as your doctor, I should already know about these!). I ask women about blood pressure problems in pregnancy and their history of oral contraceptive pill use, both of which, as we discussed previously, may be related to the development of hypertension.

It is also important to run through a series of questions concerning possible effects of hypertension. Thus, if you have had high blood pressure for a long time you might have early signs suggesting some strain on the heart, for example, chest pain or breathlessness when you walk quickly. If you have these symptoms, prompt treatment becomes more important. I also ask patients, especially older ones, about any 'funny turns' such as attacks of dizziness, weakness in the arms or legs, numbness or any other unusual symptom which might suggest that the hypertension had perhaps caused some increased hardening of the blood vessels to the brain. Again, such evidence would suggest that treatment needs to be carefully thought out. In the absence of any of these symptoms, and especially with your relatively mild hypertension, there is no need to rush into any treatment.

● I note that you have not included any questions on weight or smoking habits. Is this deliberate?

In part, yes, but I will be quizzing

you on these aspects when we discuss the plan of treatment. First, though, I need to do a physical examination.

KEY POINTS

The doctor will

✓ check family history

✓ check medical history

✓ perform a full physical examination

The physical examination

● As I did not have any of the complaints you mentioned earlier, what specific things were you looking for when you examined me?

I obviously felt your pulses; not only those in your wrists, but also in your legs and feet. I was primarily looking for any suggestion that the hypertension had caused the arteries to become harder, but I also wanted to exclude any of these rare abnormalities in the arteries that can occasionally cause hypertension. I listened very carefully to your heart, after feeling for the heartbeat through the surface of your body on your left side. If you had hypertension for a long time your heart muscles might have increased in bulk to cope with the extra pressure it had to pump against, which is another indication for a doctor that the hypertension should be treated promptly and effectively.

● You also examined my eyes – why was that necessary?

I used an ophthalmoscope, which is like an illuminated magnifying glass, to examine the blood vessels at the back of the eye. The eye is the only part of the body where we can examine the blood vessels directly. Again, if your hypertension had been fairly severe I would have seen changes in these vessels. I cannot find any problem on examining you, which indicates that the raised blood pressure has not caused you any harm.

● What other special tests do you do?

I shall test the urine sample you brought, take a blood sample and arrange for you to have an electrocardiogram.

The urine is very important as I can do a fairly simple test to check there is no protein in it. If there were I might need to look at your kidneys more closely, perhaps using a

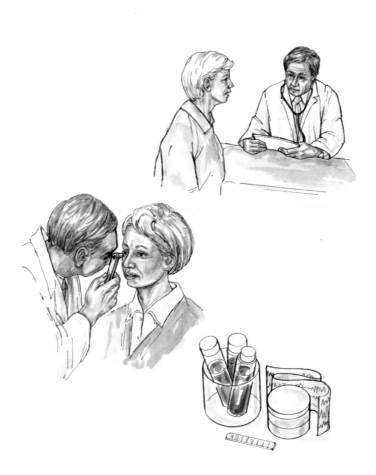

The doctor will check your family and medical history by asking a series of detailed questions. He will use an ophthalmoscope to examine the blood vessels at the back of your eye, the only part of your body where the blood vessels can be examined directly. Your heart, urine and blood will all be tested to detect the presence of hypertension.

special X-ray called an intravenous urogram, or IVU. As you know, kidney diseases can sometimes cause hypertension and also, in fact, severe hypertension can damage the kidney. It therefore makes sense to rule out these unlikely possibilities.

The blood sample will allow me to look at the balance of salts, or electrolytes as they are known. Again, if this balance were abnormal it might indicate a disturbance of kidney function. It could also provide an indication if a very rare, hormone-producing tumour were causing the hypertension.

The only other test I want to organise is an electrocardiogram or ECG. This simple, painless test records the electrical activity of the heart muscle, picked up by some metal plates placed on various parts of your body. This allows us to detect whether the heart has been put under any strain for having to pump against a very high blood pressure in the arteries. Again this is a sensible precaution to rule out any heart damage as a result of the hypertension.

With you, as with most people, nothing abnormal was found on physical examination and the urine test was fine. Hypertension can be quite a 'boring' condition for doctors, as frequently the only thing that is abnormal is the blood pressure measurement, whilst the rest of the patient is perfectly healthy!

KEY POINTS

The doctor will check

✓ pulses

✓ heart

✓ eyes

✓ urine

✓ blood

Treatment

● What sort of treatment will I need?

First, yours is the most common situation – that is, mild hypertension detected before it has done any harm – and it is reasonable to try getting the blood pressure down without drugs. However if your diastolic (lower) blood pressure were above about 105 mmHg, I would probably start drug treatment straight away.

● What non-drug options are there?

In essence, these are alterations to lifestyle which include weight reduction, salt restriction, exercise, stress limitation, though we also need to mention smoking and alcohol. Weight reduction, in your case, is most important – indeed, it is possible that your hypertension could be cured if you could get down to a normal weight.

A loss of weight of 5 kg (11lb) can reduce systolic blood pressure by 5 mmHg and diastolic blood pressure by 2.5 mmHg. There is no evidence however to suggest that weight reduction is beneficial to blood pressure in those who are not overweight, indeed it might lead to being unhealthily under weight. Losing weight is not easy and it often requires to be repeated regularly as the weight creeps up again!

● Do you have any tips for losing weight?

The most important thing is to want to lose weight. With you, for example, there is the incentive that, if losing weight brings down your blood pressure sufficiently, then you will not have to be treated with drugs. The best advice is to choose a well-balanced diet that you can stick to over a long period. One of the problems with short-term diets, particularly those which are associated with consumption of a single replacement food, such as those widely advertised in the media, is that, once you stop, old habits return and the weight increases again. We are aiming to achieve a lifetime change in dietary patterns by reducing high-calorie foods such as those that contain sugar and fats. Many patients are helped by diet sheets alone, though some like the incentive of attending a club such as Weight Watchers where you are weighed every week.

● What about salt restriction? Does that help reduce the pressure?

In many cases it can be very effective, although quite a large restriction is needed before the benefits appear.

The reduction in blood pressure achieved by a salt intake as recommended in the chapter on sodium (see page 36) is about the same as that achieved by the weight reduction discussed above. It is often the case that simultaneous reduction in weight and in sodium have a greater effect than either individually. It is probably also true that if drugs need to be used then it will be easier to control blood pressure and with a lower dose of drug if sodium intake is also restricted.

● What is the difference between salt and sodium which I have often read about in relation to blood pressure?

Salt, or more precisely, table salt, is the chemical compound sodium chloride, and it is the sodium in the compound that is relevant to blood pressure. There are a few other sources of sodium in the diet, for example, baking powder and bicarbonate of soda and reduction in their use also helps.

● I don't actually add salt to my food, so I can't see how I can reduce my intake.

Only about one-third of our salt intake comes from using salt as a condiment at the table. Most comes from processing and/or cooking food, and often we have no control over this. Many manufactured foods have large amounts of salt added. Bread, margarine, cheese, bacon and sausages are good examples. Some of these foods are basic in our diet and the salt in them cannot easily be avoided or even needs to be. Others, cheese and bacon, for example, can be eaten in smaller quantities.

Remember that many non-savoury foods on the supermarket shelves, such as breakfast cereals and biscuits, do have an unexpectedly high amount of salt. Most tinned and ready-prepared meals available are high in salt, though recently there has been a tremendous shift, as a result of consumer pressure, both to limit the amount of salt in foods and also to label the salt content on the packet.

Salt is often added in cooking, and to reduce your intake in this way requires the co-operation of the rest of your family – it is unrealistic to expect special cooking just for you! A small quantity of salt is reasonable and alternative flavourings, such as herbs and spices, should also be explored. I want to emphasise that salt is not a poison, and sensible reduction rather than total elimination is all that is necessary. The occasional kipper will not harm you, though if you succeed in reducing your salt intake you might find such food becomes too salty for your taste.

● When we talked about the causes of hypertension, you mentioned a possible protective effect of eating more potassium-containing foods to replace the sodium-containing ones. Can I make use of this for treatment purposes?

That is fairly difficult as you would need to eat very large amounts of fresh fruit, for instance, to make any impact. I would guess that if you cut down on your sodium intake your potassium intake will rise automatically, as manufactured foods are replaced by fresh foods, and it is probably the balance between the two that is important.

● Would more exercise reduce my blood pressure?

There is some evidence that regular exercise is of benefit. It is not really known how it reduces blood pressure but it seems clear that any beneficial effect only lasts as long as the exercise is undertaken regularly. Some people have achieved reductions in blood pressure by taking a longish (two-mile) walk each day. This sort of exercise often has other benefits as it can help a little in losing weight and acts as a useful opportunity to get away from the everyday stress.

Regular swimming, even at a gentle pace, is also useful exercise and has the advantage that it doesn't require good weather if you go to an indoor pool! I do not advocate strenuous exercise, especially as you are not used to it. Starting jogging or squash at your age, without a very gradual introduction, can be dangerous. I should mention that sex is perfectly safe. Despite the fact that it causes an increase in blood pressure, this is very short-lived and, in your case, would not carry any significant danger.

● Is it possible to reduce stress, and is this useful if treating high blood pressure?

This is a very difficult area and there are many differing opinions. Three methods have been tried: meditation, yoga and relaxation. The supporters of each of these methods are very enthusiastic about their success.

Most doctors have had limited experience and are probably not usefully able to comment one way or the other. There is an interesting technique called biofeedback where the patient is made aware of his or her blood pressure during normal activities and, as a result, learns which parts of their usual routine are associated with high blood pressure and thus might be avoided.

● Should I give up smoking?
An absolute yes! As said when talking about the causes of hypertension, stopping smoking will not on its own have any large effect on your blood pressure. However as a smoker your risks of developing heart attack and stroke complications from hypertension are much increased. In addition, there is very good evidence to suggest that even treating hypertension with drugs may be ineffective in reducing these complications in smokers. Put another way, high blood pressure increases your risk of heart attack as does smoking, the two in combination increase the risk to a much greater extent than each acting independently.

● Do I have to give up alcohol as well? I like the occasional drink.
There is no need to give up the occasional drink. However alcohol can be quite fattening – a gin and tonic can contain as many calories as a slice of chocolate cake – and obesity is a risk factor for hypertension.

Excessive alcohol intake is becoming increasingly recognised as an important factor in the development of hypertension, and might account for up to a quarter of all cases of hypertension. A reduction in alcohol level can achieve similar reductions in blood pressure to that obtained by weight reduction. Your maximum intake should be one 'standard' drink (half a pint of beer, one measure of spirit, or a small glass of wine) per day. The benefits from alcohol reduction may take a few months to show themselves as the body 'recovers' from a long-term problem. Reduction in alcohol has many other health benefits both in the short term and the longer term. Compared to giving up smoking or losing weight, you may find it easier to reduce alcohol consumption, and so perhaps it should be the first target for action.

● How long will you try these non-drug measures before deciding whether they are sufficient in my case?
If these measures have not been successful in three months, we will probably need to consider drug treatment. If they work, however, then you may need no other form of treatment, providing you maintain the change in lifestyle.

I will ask the practice nurse to check your blood pressure every month for the next three months to see how you progress.

● My friend's doctor gave him drug treatment first. Why?

If the blood pressure is very high, or there is any suggestion of heart or blood vessel damage from the hypertension, then drugs are really needed. Furthermore, the response to drugs tends to be more predictable; salt restriction or weight loss for instance do not work with everyone. It is also easier to tailor the dose of drugs to give the right amount. With changes in lifestyle, we are really making educated guesses. For example, I do not know exactly how much weight you need to lose. Finally, the changes in lifestyle demanded may be too difficult to adhere to, and often a lot of my advice to patients is ignored! Against these disadvantages there are the gains of cost-saving (including prescription charges) by not using drugs, and the anxiety that long-term drug treatment may have harmful side-effects. It is a difficult decision, but in your case it is probably worth trying without drugs first.

● I have now had three months treatment without drugs, but with little reduction in blood pressure. The next step, I gather, is to start drug treatment. What are the different types of drugs available, and how do they act?

There are a large number of different drugs, but they fall into a smallish number of different groups or classes of drugs. Within each class there are a number of available drugs. The different classes reduce blood pressure in different ways, whereas the drugs within a particular class act in roughly the same way.

The first group are the *diuretics*. These drugs are sometimes called 'water tablets' because the main action noticed by the patient is to increase the volume of urine passed. They actually work by increasing the amount of sodium salt passed in the urine, and the extra water passed just accompanies the salt. There are many different diuretics used in the treatment of blood pressure. The commonest are called *thiazides*. They are often used alone in mild hypertension, and are frequently combined with other drugs in more severe cases.

Their one possible problem is that they cause a loss of potassium as well as sodium in the urine. This is easily combated by either giving extra potassium or by adding another diuretic which retains potassium. Not all doctors agree that it is necessary to add potassium to a thiazide diuretic and many believe that a diet with plenty of fresh fruit is often sufficient. If you are taking this type of drug it is sensible is to have the concentration of potassium in your blood checked from time to time. Diuretics are normally given as a single daily dose in the morning (as soon as you wake up) to get the increase in urine output over with as quickly as possible in the day.

The second, widely used group are called the *beta blockers*. This group of drugs has two main actions in reducing blood pressure. They reduce both the heart rate (the number of times the heart beats per minute), as well as the amount of blood pumped out of the heart by each beat. Thus their overall effect is to reduce the amount of blood pumped by the heart into the arteries, and this is in turn reduces the pressure.

There are at least a dozen different beta blockers available, with one of the differences between them being their length of action. Some beta blockers have to be taken three times a day to maintain an effect, whereas others, such as *atenolol* ('Tenormin'), *betaxolol* ('Kerlone') or *metoprolol* ('Betaloc') can be given as a single daily dose in the morning. Tablets are available that combine a diuretic and beta blockers. This simplifies treatment, but reduces the flexibility of dose.

Until fairly recently these were the commonest groups of drugs with which to start treatment, but two other groups are becoming increasingly used, particularly when diuret-ics and beta blockers either prove ineffective or cause side-effects.

The first are *calcium channel blockers*, for example *nifedipine* ('Adalat'). They work by acting on the heart and also on the muscle in the walls of the arteries. Their effect on the arteries is to widen the small blood vessels, a property known as vasodilating. Calcium channel blockers are only one of a number of groups that have this artery widening or vasodilating property. In the past, however, these other vasodilator drugs were often used when diuretics and beta blockers were insufficient.

The second new group are called *ACE inhibitors; captopril* ('Capoten') and *enalapril* ('Innovace') were the first of the available drugs in this group. These actually block the production of an enzyme which is thought to be overproduced in hypertension, and on theoretical grounds, represent a sound basis for treatment.

There are other groups of drugs but as they tend to be used only if one or combinations of the above drugs do not work, there is perhaps no need to discuss them further here.

● Why does the same drug have more than one name, and which, if any, of the names is it important for me to remember?

It is important that you know the names and dosages of any drug you are taking for hypertension, and you should carry a card with you which gives these details in case of emergency. All drugs have at least two names. The first is the approved name, which is the name of the chemical in the tablet. The second is the trade name that the manufacturers use. Often the latter are easier to remember and even spell! The problem is that the same drug is sometimes marketed by more than one company, and hence can have a number of different trade names. If you stick to noting only the approved name it probably gives less grounds for confusion.

● How does the doctor decide which drug to start with?
Most doctors would actually choose between a diuretic and a beta blocker first, then, if these failed, move on to a combination of the two before adding one of the other groups of drugs. The effect of diuretics is not really enhanced by increasing the dose, whereas, with beta blockers, a small dose can be tried first which can be followed by a larger dose if there is no response. In some patients there may be some particular medical reason why neither diuretics nor beta blockers are the appropriate way to begin treatment, and we would need to use one of the other drugs. The aim is to get blood pressure controlled on the smallest dose of the smallest number of drugs possible. Occasionally, though, it is necessary in some patients to combine two, three or even four drugs to get the blood pressure controlled. I should emphasise, however, that this is exceedingly rare.

● I realise it is important never to miss a dose, but if I do, should I take double the dose next time?
First, it is important that you take the drugs exactly as prescribed. Having said that, we are all human, and it is very easy to forget, especially when you are taking a drug more than once a day. If this is happening regularly it is sensible to tell your doctor and perhaps a simpler regimen can be found. Never take more than the prescribed dose of any drug without seeking medical advice. The occasional missed dose will not put you in any immediate danger!

● What about side-effects? I suppose I am not unusual in being worried about these drugs being harmful?
Anxiety about side-effects is very common, and indeed, justified when you consider that we are asking you to take drugs for a condition which has no symptoms. Doctors are very wary of making the treatment worse than the disease!

If you suspect that you are having a side-effect from the drug, always seek medical advice before stopping it, preferably in person, though if a side-effect occurs very shortly after starting a new drug, then it might be reasonable to telephone for advice.

I think it is fair to say that many of the drugs that were widely used 15 to 20 years ago did cause side-effects in many patients – most noticeably dizziness when the patient stood up. The drugs used today are much better tolerated. Diuretics, apart from the inconvenience of increasing urine output, only rarely cause any problems and are indeed very safe drugs. I have already mentioned potassium loss, which is easily spotted and remedied or prevented.

Beta blockers do have some side-effects in some patients. The effects tend to be different with different beta blockers. A few patients complain of feeling tired and have no energy. Often this improves spontaneously without changing the treatment, though sometimes it is worth trying a different beta blocker or even changing to another group of drugs. Some patients on certain beta blockers may cause wheezing in people who have lung problems, such as asthma or bronchitis, but there are other beta blocker drugs that do not have this side-effect and can be used instead.

Otherwise, all the drugs I have mentioned are generally tolerated very well. Any patient can have an allergic reaction to a particular drug and develop a rash or something similar, but these reactions are not peculiar to blood pressure drugs.

KEY POINTS

✓ Non-drug options
- reduce weight
- restrict salt intake
- increase exercise
- lower stress
- lower alcohol intake

✓ Smoking and hypertension reinforce each other's bad effects
- kick the habit

✓ Drug options
- diuretics – can cause potassium loss
- beta blockers
- calcium channel blockers
- ACE inhibitors

The future

● How often do I need to have my blood pressure measured?

The short answer is as often as is necessary.

Unless your blood pressure is very high, once a month is probably sufficient, and then I can give you a further month's supply of treatment.

This pattern will then continue until your blood pressure has remained steady at a normal level for three months or so. Then we can move to checks every two, or even, three months.

● What level of blood pressure do you aim for in treatment?

I would like your diastolic blood pressure to remain below 90 mmHg.

However if your blood pressure had remained below this level for some months on the same treatment, and then you had one raised reading, I would not necessarily rush in to change anything.

● For how long will I need treatment?

I have some patients whose hypertension often 'cures itself' after a few months or even years of treatment. Treatment itself only reduces blood pressure, it doesn't actually attack the cause, and therefore to talk of cure is misleading. I suspect that many of these 'cured' patients have either managed to lose weight or have become less stressed. For most treatment continues for life, though with a simple drug regimen, taking the tablet becomes as much a part of everyday existence as brushing your teeth. Indeed, it is very important not to consider yourself as ill just because you need to take daily treatment. It is a preventative measure that will help to keep you in good health.

● Will hypertension affect my life insurance risk?

Unfortunately, yes, and you have to

expect higher premiums. Before completing a proposal form, it is important to ask companies if they add any loading for hypertension and you can then choose the most generous option. If your hypertension remains mild and your blood pressure is well-controlled on treatment, this reduces the extra loading. The life insurance companies will also look more favourably on you if you are a non-smoker and not overweight.

● Does my hypertension prevent my participating in normal activities?

The short answer is no. Reasonable exertion as we discussed earlier is perfectly safe and, indeed, useful. Sexual intercourse is not harmful. Similarly, there is no bar to your driving a car. Air travel is also perfectly acceptable, but obviously if you travel abroad you must take sufficient tablets for your stay.

● Do women with hypertension have to avoid becoming pregnant?

Normal pregnancy can have a hypertensive effect: hypertension can affect the growing baby and the drugs used for hypertension could be dangerous. Having said that, however, pregnancy is safe, provided that the mother's blood pressure is carefully monitored throughout pregnancy and labour.

● One last point – I was very upset when you found my blood pressure was high when you first measured it, but from all the discussions we have had, I am now pleased that it was discovered. I know that I will probably have to take drugs for the foreseeable future, but in many ways I feel reassured that I am now protected.

I am glad to hear that. If you stick to the advice and treatment I have given you there is every reason to think that your condition will give you little trouble.

KEY POINTS

✓ Patients with hypertension need their blood pressure checking every month

✓ Hypertension is a condition not a disease, though it can be for life

✓ Even if you have hypertension you can still lead a normal life

Sodium content of common foods

The sodium content of the foods listed in the tables on the following pages should provide a guide to putting together a sensible diet.

For the sake of simplicity the amount of sodium is expressed in milligrams (mg) per 100 grams of the food (approximately 3.5 ounces) rather than per typical portion. For someone with raised blood pressure, a reasonable average daily intake would be between 2 and 2.5 grams of sodium.

The contents list printed on packaged food might give the sodium content as salt (sodium chloride).

As a rough guide slightly less than half the weight of table salt is sodium and so the recommended intake of 2 to 2.5 grams is equivalent to an intake of 5 to 6 grams of salt.

A number of general points:

● Even without adding salt as a condiment there are many foods with a very high salt content

● Raw fruit and vegetables have negligible amounts of sodium. It is the processing and cooking that are responsible for most of our intake

● The levels are given as a guide only. For example, there are clear differences between different margarines, cheeses, etc.

FOOD GROUP

SODIUM CONTENT (mg/100 grams)

Cereals and cereal products

All-Bran		900
Biscuits:	chocolate	160
	cream crackers	610
	digestive: chocolate	450
	plain	600
	oatcakes	1230
	shortbread	230
Bread:	brown	540
	Hovis	600
	malt	280
	white	520
	white toasted	650
Cornflakes: Kellogg's		1110
Custard powder		320
Muesli:	with no added sugar	47
Poppadums: fried in vegetable oil		2420
Pasta:	macaroni, uncooked	11
	noodles, uncooked	180
	spaghetti: canned	420
	white, uncooked	3
	wholemeal, uncooked	130
Pizza		570
Porridge, with water		560
Ready Brek		12
Rice:	brown, uncooked	3
	savoury, uncooked	1440
	white, uncooked	4
Rice Krispies		1260
Shredded Wheat		8
Weetabix		270
Wheat flour: brown		4
	bread making	3
	self-raising	360

Milk and milk products

Cheese:	Cheddar	670
	cream	300

	fromage frais, plain	31
	processed	1320
	spread	1060
Condensed milk, sweetened		150
Cream:	clotted	18
	double	37
	Dream Topping	70
	single	49
	dried skimmed milk	550
Flavoured milk		61
Human milk, colostrum		47
Ice cream, dairy, vanilla		69
Skimmed milk, average		54
Semi-skimmed milk, average		55
Soya milk, plain		32
Whole milk, average		55
Yoghurt, low fat, plain		83
Egg:	whole, uncooked	140
	white, uncooked	190
	yolk, uncooked	50
	fried	160
Omelette, plain		1030

Fats

Butter	750
Corn oil	Trace
Lard	2
Margarine	800
Olive oil	Trace
Spread, very low fat	1050

Cakes and pastries

Currant buns		230
Doughnuts, ring		230
Fruit cake, plain		250
Jam tarts, short pastry		230
Pastry:	flaky, cooked	460
	short, cooked	480
	wholemeal, cooked	410
Scones		770
Sponge cake		350

Swiss roll, chocolate	350

Puddings
Bread puddings	310
Cheesecake	160
Custard, milk	81
Fruit crumble	64
Instant dessert powder	1100
Jelly	5
Pancakes, made with milk	53
Rice pudding, canned	50
Treacle tart	360
Trifle	53

Sugar, preserves and snacks
Chocolate, milk	120
Fruit gums	64
Honey	11
Jam	16
Mars Bars	150
Mincemeat	140
Potato crisps	1070
Sugar: demerara	6
white	Trace
Syrup, golden	270
Toffee, mixed	320

Vegetables
Beans: baked, canned	530
french, boiled	8
runner, uncooked	Trace
Beetroot, boiled	110
Brussels sprouts, boiled	2
Cabbage: uncooked	5
boiled in salted water	100
Carrots: old, uncooked	25
canned	370
Celery, uncooked	60
Cucumber, uncooked	3
Lentils, uncooked	12
Mushrooms, uncooked	5

Onions:	uncooked	3
	boiled	2
	fried	4
	pickled	450
Peas:	fresh, uncooked	1
	tinned	250
Potatoes:	old, uncooked	7
	old, baked in skin	12
	old, chipped, retail	35
	old, french fries	310
	new, boiled	9
	new, canned	250
	waffles	430
Processed peas, canned		380
Spinach, boiled		120
Swedes, uncooked		15
Sweetcorn:	baby, canned	1140
	on-the-cob	1
Tomatoes:	canned	39
	uncooked	9
	puree	240
Watercress, uncooked		49

Fruit and nuts

Apples:	eating	3
	cooking: uncooked	2
	stewed	4
Apricots:	fresh	14
	canned in syrup	10
Bananas		1
Cherries:	uncooked	1
	glacé	27
Chestnuts		11
Coconut, desiccated		28
Currants		14
Figs, dried, uncooked		62
Fruit salad, tinned, syrup		3
Grapes, black		2
Lemons, whole		5
Melons		8
Mixed nuts		300

Nectarines		1
Olives (in brine)		2250
Oranges		5
Peaches, fresh		1
Pears, English, eating		3
Peanuts:	plain	2
	dry roasted	790
Peanut butter		350
Prunes, canned in juice		18
Raisins, dried		60
Sultana, dried		19

Meat, poultry and game products

Bacon:	fat, uncooked	560
	lean, uncooked	1870
Beef:	burgers, frozen, fried	880
	uncooked, average	33
	rump steak, uncooked	51
	silverside, salted, boiled	1000
Black pudding		1210
Chicken:	boiled	82
	roast	81
Chilli con carne		250
Duck, roast		96
Ham and pork, chopped, canned		1090
Kidney, sheep, fried		270
Lamb, cooked, average		56
Liver, calf, fried		170
Meat paste		740
Mince:	uncooked	86
	stewed	320
Pork chops, grilled, lean		84
Salami		1850
Sausage:	pork, fried	1050
	grilled	1000
Turkey, roast		57

Fish

Cockles		3520
Cod:	uncooked, fillets	77
	fried	100

grilled	91
Crab: boiled	370
canned	550
Fish fingers, grilled	380
Fish paste	600
Haddock: fresh, steamed	120
fried	160
smoked, steamed	1220
Kippers, baked	990
Lemon sole, fried	140
Lobster, boiled	330
Mussels, boiled	210
Plaice: steamed	120
fried	220
Salmon: fresh, steamed	110
tinned	570
smoked	1880
Sardines, tinned	700
Shrimps: frozen, shell removed	375
canned, drained	980
Trout, steamed	88

Beverages

Coca-cola	8
Cocoa powder	950
Coffee and chicory essence	65
Coffeemate	200
Complan powder	1800
Drinking chocolate powder	250
Lucozade	28
Malted milk, Horlicks	460
Orange: drink, undiluted	21
juice	10
Tea	Trace
Tomato juice	230

Alcoholic beverages

Bitter, draught	12
Pale ale, bottled	10
Strong ale	15
Stout, bottled	23

| Wine: | red | 10 |
| | white | 4 |

Soups, sauces and miscellaneous foods

Bovril	4800
Cream of chicken soup, canned	460
Curry powder	450
French dressing	930
Instant soup powder	3440
Marmite	4500
Minestrone soup, dried	5600
Nutmeg	16
Oxo cubes	10300
Pepper, black	44
Pickle	1700
Tomato ketchup	1120
Tomato soup: canned	460
dried	4040
Salad cream	1040
Salt, table	38700
Soy sauce	5720
Vegetable soup, canned	500

The data in these tables are adapted from the standard publication of nutrient content of common foods: *Chemical Composition of Foods* published by HMSO in 1991.

Drugs

There are numerous drugs currently used to treat high blood pressure, grouped into four main classes. The differences between drugs in any one category are small though duration of action is an important consideration. Thus some beta blockers have a long life of action and can be given once a day whereas others need to be given two or more times. In addition, however, some quick acting drugs can be manufactured to have a slow release to give a longer life. They are often given the suffix LA (long acting) or SR (slow release).

TYPE OF DRUG	CHEMICAL NAME	TRADE NAME*
Diuretics		
Thiazides	bendrofluazide	Aprinox
		Berkozide
	chlorothiazide	Saluric
	chlorthalidone	Hygroton
	cyclopenthiazide	Navidrex
	hydrochlorothiazide	Esidrex
		Hydrosaluric
	hydroflumethiazide	Hydrenox
	indapamide	Natrilix
	mefruside	Baycaron
	metolazone	Metenix 5
	polythiazide	Nephril
	xipamide	Diurexan

Potassium sparing	amiloride	As a group this class
	triamterene	of drugs is unlikely to
	spironolactone	be used on its own
		and is normally
		combined with a
		thiazide
Thiazide plus potassium	Various combinations normally with 'K' at end	
	of name e.g. Centyl K	
Thiazide plus potassium	A large number exist combining one from each	
sparing	of these two categories e.g. Dyazide	
	(triamterene and hydrochlorothiazide)	

Beta blockers	acebutolol	Sectral
	atenolol	Antipressan
		Tenormin
	betaxolol	Kerlone
	bisoprolol	Emcor
		Monocor
	celiprolol	Celectol
	metoprolol	Arbralene
		Betaloc
		Lopressor
	nadolol	Corgard
	oxprenolol	Trasicor
	pindolol	Visken
	propanolol	Inderal and many
		others
	sotalol	Sotacor
		Beta-Cardone
	timolol	Blocardren and others
Beta blocker/	This list is almost endless of drugs which	
diuretic combinations	combine within the same tablet a diuretic,	
	normally a thiazide, with a beta blocker. Some	
	formulations combine a thiazide and a	
	potassium sparing diuretic with a beta blocker	

ACE Inhibitors	captropril	Acepril
		Capoten
	enalapril	Innovace
	fosinopril	Staril
	lisinopril	Carace

		Zestril
	perindopril	Coversyl
	quinapril	Accupro
	ramipril	Tritace
	trandolapril	Gopten
		Odrik
ACE Inhibitor/thiazide combination	Many of the ACE inhibitors listed above are also available combined with a thiazide, e.g. Capozide (captopril and hydrochlorothiazide)	

Calcium-channel blockers	amlodipine	Istin
	diltiazem	Dilzem
		Tildiem
	felodipine	Plendil
	isradipine	Prescal
	nicardipine	Cardene
	nifedipine	Adalat and others

*This list is based on drugs listed in the ABPI Data Sheet Compendium for 1994/95 and though reasonably comprehensive may not include all drugs in a particular class.

Glossary

This glossary explains the meaning of the most frequently used clinical and related terms connected with the diagnosis and treatment of high blood pressure (hypertension).

accelerated hypertension: a rather old fashioned term to describe severe hypertension, which was difficult to treat. Fallen into disuse given the availability of modern effective drugs

ACE inhibitors: a group of drugs which work by blocking the enzyme acetyl cholinesterase. Increasingly used in all classes of hypertension

albumin: a protein, made by the liver, which can leak into the urine if there is damage to the kidneys. Such damage can be caused, amongst other disorders, by severe inadequately treated hypertension

albuminuria: abnormal presence of albumin in the urine

aneroid: a type of sphygmomanometer, which is very portable and often used for home visits

antihypertensive: a drug which is capable of lowering blood pressure

arteriole: the small arteries which are important in the normal regulation of blood pressure

arteriosclerosis: often referred to as hardening of the arteries and describes the changes to the structure of the walls of arteries caused by prolonged untreated hypertension. The artery becomes hardened and this can affect blood supply

artery: name of any blood vessel that supplies blood to a part of the body (see vein)

bd (or **bid**): abbreviation of a Latin term meaning twice a day, used in writing prescriptions

beta blocker: probably the most widely used of all classes of anti-hypertensive drugs, they work by essentially reducing the amount of blood pumped out by the heart during each beat

blister pack: a convenient method of packaging tablets that need to be taken once a day. Each pack typically contains a four-week supply of tablets each in its own foil or similar blister, labelled with the day of the week. It is a useful means of ensuring compliance with regular medication

body mass index (BMI): a widely used measure of obesity, obtained by dividing weight by height squared. If weight is in kilograms and height is in metres the BMI is normally in the range 25–30

brittle: an infrequently used term to describe the situation where it is difficult to control a patient's blood pressure without frequent changes of therapy

calcium channel blocker: a group of antihypertensive drugs that work by causing vasodilation (*see below*)

cerebral arteries: arteries that supply the brain and are vulnerable to damage by prolonged untreated hypertension

combination therapy: used to describe the common situation of treating hypertension with more than one drug, which might be combined in a single tablet (e.g. a diuretic and a beta blocker)

compliance: an indication of how far instructions for treatment are adhered to. In conditions such as hypertension which do not cause symptoms it is often difficult to maintain complete compliance even with the most motivated patient

contra-indication: any state that should prevent a particular therapy being commenced. A list of these are provided in the data sheet for each drug. For example asthma is a contra-indication for the use of some beta blockers, since they could make it worse

coronary arteries: arteries that supply the heart muscle and are vulnerable to damage from hypertension

coronary thrombosis: *see* myocardial infarction

cuff: describes the rubber bag covered in material, wrapped round the arm during the measurement of blood pressure by a sphygmomanometer

data sheet: gives the details about each drug. A data sheet has to be issued by the manufacturers to inform the prescriber. They are gathered together in books, and the prescribing doctor may well consult such a source during a consultation to check details about dose, contraindications or possible side-effects

diastole: the phase during the cycle of the heart when it is filling with blood and the pressure in the arteries is at its lowest

diastolic blood pressure: the arterial pressure recorded during diastole

die: : Latin for day and used in prescriptions (*see bd, tds*)

dipstick: used to describe the widely available plastic strips which have small squares of impregnated chemicals used to dip into a sample of urine to obtain a rapid assessment, for example, of an abnormally high level of albumin

diuretic: a very widely used class of antihypertensive drugs which work by increasing the amount of sodium passed out in the urine. Often inappropriately called water tablets – the increased amount of water passed is

secondary to the increased level of sodium

ECG: *see* electrocardiograph

EKG: American term for ECG

electrocardiograph: a widely used test of heart function obtained by placing pads on the surface of the body and recording the heart's electrical activity. In hypertension useful for measuring any increased thickness in the left ventricle (*see below*) and any evidence of coronary artery disease

electrolyte balance: refers to the measurement in the blood of the concentration of sodium, potassium and chloride. May be used to monitor some therapy such as diuretics where potassium loss might be important to detect

heart attack: lay term for myocardial infarction

heart rate: measurement of the time the heart contracts per minute, normally obtained by feeling the pulse at the wrist, although if the heart is irregular it may be more accurately measured by listening to the heart with a stethoscope or using an ECG

hypertension: medical term for an abnormally and persistently raised blood pressure

hypertensive: an individual with hypertension, or an agent such as a drug that might induce hypertension

hypertrophy: enlargement in bulk, in relation to hypertension. Refers to enlargement of the left ventricle or main chamber of the heart. If left ventricular hypertrophy is demonstrated, this indicates that the excessive rise in blood pressure has caused the heart to increase in muscle bulk to overcome this

hypotension: abnormally low blood pressure which might result from over treatment of hypertension or may rarely result from a specific disorder

iatrogenic: refers to a problem resulting from medical intervention, for example the side-effects of drugs. In a common disorder such as hypertension there is always the anxiety that the risks from iatrogenic problems can counter the potential benefits from effective treatment

kidney: the organ in the body responsible for maintaining electrolyte balance. Many antihypertensive drugs work by direct action on the kidney. Chronic diseases of the kidneys may result in hypertension and hypertension itself can damage the kidneys, so setting up a vicious cycle

labile: blood pressure that is normally very variable and even in the same 24-hour period might swing between being definitely normal and definitely abnormal. May not require therapy

left ventricle: the largest chamber in the heart which stores the blood and then pumps it out during systole. May be damaged by prolonged untreated hypertension (*see* hypertrophy)

mane: Latin for in the morning, used in prescriptions. Diuretics (*see above*) are usefully taken in the morning so that the excess urine loss that results might be finished sufficiently early in the day to provide the minimum inconvenience

myocardial infarction: medical term for heart attack. Used to describe the damage caused when part of the heart muscle, typically of the left ventricle, loses its blood supply temporarily as a result of a localised blockage of one of the coronary arteries. Hypertension is one of the main risk factors for this. Indeed the prevention of myocardial infarction and stroke is the reason for treating hypertension

nocte: Latin for night, used in prescriptions to indicate medication taken once daily at night-time.

Compliance is better at night than in the morning

normotensive: normal blood pressure

obesity: medical term for being overweight for height

ophthalmoscope: illuminated magnifying item of medical equipment, routinely used in monitoring the care of a patient with hypertension to check for retinal artery damage

pharmacological: relating to drugs. For example in hypertension both non-pharmacological (e.g. low salt diet) and pharmacological treatments (e.g. diuretics) have been proposed

postural hypotension: a fall in blood pressure on standing from the sitting or lying position. May be a consequence of therapy and lead to dizziness on rising

potassium: an electrolyte which may be important in hypertension. Use of diuretics may cause excessive loss of potassium from the body though some diuretics ('potassium sparing diuretics') do not have this side-effect. Potassium is also naturally available in foods and is used in salt substitutes.

proteinuria: excess excretion of protein, normally albumin, by the kidneys. A very sensitive test of kidney damage

pulse: the impulse of systole felt over arteries at sites near the surface of the body, e.g. at the wrist

pulse pressure: the difference between systolic and diastolic pressure, the greater the value the more pronounced the impulse felt when feeling the pulse. Often much greater in the elderly

qds (qid): abbreviation of a Latin term meaning four times a day, used in writing prescriptions

renal: refers to the kidney

renal artery: the main artery supplying the kidney. Very rarely a narrowing of this artery might be the cause of hypertension, which can then be cured by surgery

retina: the back of the eye which, with its detailed blood supply, is visible through an ophthalmoscope. Useful in monitoring hypertension as it provides the best site for visualising the effect of hypertension on arterioles

retinopathy: describes an abnormality of the retina. There are a number of disorders that can affect the retina but there are distinct patterns that are discernible in hypertensive retinopathy

salt: in normal use refers to table salt or sodium chloride *(see* sodium)

salt substitute: a condiment which contains non-sodium containing compounds such as potassium chloride which may be of some value in achieving dietary sodium restriction

screening: represents the detection of a disorder before it has become apparent to the subject. Hypertension is an excellent example as in the vast majority of cases there are no symptoms and without screening it would not have been detected

sodium: an important electrolyte involved in hypertension. Excessive sodium intake as sodium chloride or other compounds such as sodium bicarbonate (bicarb of soda) might be important in leading to hypertension; conversely sodium restriction might be a useful therapy

sphygmomanometer: the most widely used instrument for measuring blood pressure

stroke: used to describe problem caused by temporary interruption of blood supply to the brain which lasts for a sufficiently long period to lead to brain damage. Although often short lived the damage may be irreversible and its prevention is the most important justification for treatment of hypertension

systole: the phase during the cycle of the heart when it pumps out the blood and the pressure in the arteries is at its highest

systolic blood pressure: the arterial pressure recorded during systole

tds (*tid)***: abbreviation of a Latin term meaning three times a day, used in writing prescriptions

thiazide: the most commonly prescribed class of diuretics in hypertension; taking them might lead to excessive loss of potassium

urea: a compound resulting from the chemical breakdown of proteins which is passed by the kidneys in the urine as the means of getting rid of excess nitrogen from the body. Often measured in the blood the same time as electrolytes (U&E's). Will be raised in the blood if there is severe kidney damage or if there had been excessive water loss due to, say, over-use of diuretics.

urine collection (24 hour): it may be necessary to collect all urine passed in a 24-hour period either to measure electrolyte or protein passed by the kidneys

vasoconstriction: the narrowing of the diameter of arteries and arterioles by contraction of muscles in their walls, or importance in the development of hypertension

vasodilation: the widening of the diameter of arteries and arterioles by relaxing of muscles in their walls. Drugs which act as vasodilators can be effective in reducing blood pressure

vein: name of any blood vessel that takes blood away from a part of the body (*see* artery), not involved in hypertension

water tablet: *see* diuretic

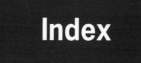

Index